MW01714411

Drowning Lessons

Drowning Lessons

MAUREEN SCOTT HARRIS

PEDLAR PRESS | TORONTO

Copyright © Maureen Scott Harris 2004

ALL RIGHTS RESERVED. No part of this book may be reproduced or transmitted in any form or by any means whatsoever without written permission from the publisher, except by a reviewer, who may quote brief passages in a review. For information, write Pedlar Press at PO Box 26, Station P, Toronto Ontario M5S 2S6 Canada.

ACKNOWLEDGEMENTS
The publisher wishes to thank the Canada Council for the Arts and the Ontario Arts Council for their generous support of our publishing program.

Edited for the press by Barry Dempster.

CANADIAN CATALOGUING IN PUBLICATION DATA

Harris, Maureen, 1943-
Drowning lessons / Maureen Scott Harris.

Poems.
ISBN 0-9732140-8-2

I. Title.

PS8565.A64885D76 2004 C811 .54 C2004-903810-9

First Edition

COVER PHOTOGRAPH Joan Kaufman
DESIGN Zab Design & Typography, Winnipeg
TYPEFACE (Headings) Introducing *Rubber Bit*, designed by Zab

Printed in Canada

The Canada Council for the Arts since 1957 | Le Conseil des Arts du Canada depuis 1957

Ontario Arts Council
Conseil des Arts de l'Ontario

For Peter,

For Jessica, and Katharine

and

For Stuart

Contents

Mother Cupboard

everyone has a life like this

full of packing cases with straw and
paper from around the china spilling out
on scarred linoleum
when the telephone rings and

it's never possible to see everything
in its place or a place for whatever
you're holding in your hand, or were,
before the phone rang and you ran for it

and whatever it was has settled so well
wherever you put it you no longer know
what it was or why you were standing there
hauling things out of packing cases

dripping straw and paper you stand bare-
handed, wondering where you've been
who called

Family Pastimes

The chairs wait so patiently assembled in groups in the rain.
The smallest must have clambered onto the picnic table
where it sits still now. The barbecue is open-mouthed and
one square white table leans against the peeling fence.
The blue rocking horse stares. Its solid blue eyes ignore
the upturned yellow wading pool stained with wet leaves.
Beside empty flower pots the children's plastic chairs
have turned their backs on each other. Something has been left out.

No one sits in the canvas lawn chair beside a tin table with
a half-filled glass on it. No one crosses the yard
to the picnic table. The chairs do not move.
In the spaces among them wind and weeds.

The emptiness of objects, of memory.
So many things. No one has turned or returned
to wipe the furniture clean and dry, rake up old sticks and leaves,
compile conversations, disassemble histories. Slowly
the table sags. Chairs surrender to the lawn. The fence slips
sideways as light splinters across the yard.
The slight wind murmurs, pushing at the fence, waving
leaves in the rain, moving through.

Twilight

All over the city at this hour
the sky dims and lights come on.
In the dusk women stand in doorways,
at windows, waiting. There are babies
with them. *Let the hour pass* they say
a door open. Make a breeze stir.
Women stand holding babies and murmur
into the thick slow silence.
They inhale the sweet scent of baby skin.
Women stare into the dusk holding babies
and wait for sleep, conversation,
the second coming, anything at all
to draw in-here and out-there
together.

I Spy Mother Cupboard

Here comes Mother Cupboard
arms spread wide to scoop us up
her breasts overflowing
with milk and honey.

She sings aloud in the kitchen,
carols of yeast and cinnamon,
and our spirits rise with the dough.
Her table warbles with pleasure

under its burden of feasts.
We flutter round it, mouths
open, begging to be fed,
and with a snap of her fingers

raspberries leap whole and glowing
into a bowl of cream.
Every spoonful whispers *love, love*.
From the pockets of her flowered housecoat

she hands us chocolate, apples,
raisins and fresh bread,
all the comforts we need.
Mother Cupboard's warm hands

nestle us into her cupboard heart
where we're lulled by its muffled beat,
dreaming dreams to fatten on.
The real taste, we know, is her.

Mother Cupboard's Dream

Tired, so tired, Mother Cupboard shuts her cupboard heart and lies her weary bones down to sleep. She wants only the dark and the silence, but her thoughts twist and turn.

The old nightmare surfaces — the cupboard is bare, open mouths cluster around her. Whining and begging for food, they chew at her sleeves, glide their tongues across her knees. She shudders, slides into a sleep riddled by the yap of her empty heart.

She dreams the cupboard is full of pickled children and she is ravenous.

The Particulars

The particulars peel away day by day,
words forgotten or fumbled for,
things she does falling unnoticed at her feet.

He stares at her as if she is someone
he used to pass on the street.
Looking more closely it's himself he glimpses
in her unseeing eyes.

So much is given away, is never grasped.
If only she wasn't taking pieces of him with her —
the story they'd shared of a perfect past
the two of them walking hand in hand along a street.
She clutches and he wants to pull away.

Shavings of bone, patches of skin, a knuckle
float into that tunnel she stares down,
leaving him imperfect, stuttering, unable
to stop himself falling away even as he watches.
He could disown her now, stand up and leave
as if she'd never contained a trace of him.

Cut off a finger, cut out a tongue, stitch
eyes shut, it is all no good, she is still
there, this old woman who appeared one day
wearing some shreds of his mother's face.

Flowers for My Mother

A door opens onto a winter street spilling light and warmth.
I come out of the dark my arms full of flowers, my hands cold.
I arrive breathless, pulling my face together,
becoming solid. The flowers blaze —

Hearing the crunch of snow, feeling my fingertips burn, I remember
other doorways spilling light, smells of cinnamon and meatloaf,
and I'm not myself, who I was
licked into shape, stumbling into the light.

I'm here. Breathless. My arms alight
with red poinsettia and white chrysanthemum.
Flowers blood-scarlet and white as prairie snow flare in the dark.
Those days dimming toward winter, the muteness of falling snow.

The silence of flowers thickens my tongue, I cannot
say I hate you, I cannot say I love you. *Nothing is done with*
I want to say. Close the door on the dark and the dark's still
there. *See me.* I'm on both sides of the door.

But I'm wordless, blinking into the light, breathless
at crossing the threshold, ghosts
everywhere, darkness or light, it's cold and
here are these flowers for you, red and white in the winter night.

Looking at Photographs of My Daughters

I've taken so many pictures of you from behind,
mesmerized first by the way your hair
spiralled around your perfect baby skulls
mirroring snailshell, galaxy, this
new universe I'd fallen into.
Year after year I looked at you looking away.

But here's a picture I'd forgotten:
foggy weather and you stand, backs to me
and larger than I knew, on an apron of
rock at the sea's edge.
I can't see your expressions, I don't know
how you feel, there, where
the waves are dark and larger than life.
There's nothing between ocean and sky and
my fear falling into the picture.

Standing behind you I hold my heart tight, not
letting out the fear:
that you will be swept away,
that you will turn and see me, hand
across my mouth, eyes round and terrified and

I want you to be happy.

Standing behind you I don't have to see myself
reflected in your eyes, the three of us so muddled
in my heart I can't skim us apart.
I want to be perfect, better
than my mother. My gaze is
the weight on your shoulders. It stiffens your necks.

Sunday Morning We Wake to Rain

Downstairs K. is practising the piano
and little spurts of sound drift up
accompanied by patter of rain, shrill
starling whistles, the occasional
lick of traffic on wet roads,
streetcars rumbling a block away.

Time asks nothing of us.

Rain beads the window, hangs
from each hawthorn branch
like a silver bauble.

The oak in the backyard is half-bare,
riddled by the squirrels' foraging.
Even as I watch
leaves come loose
in handfuls.

Early Childhood Education

1

The girl must not
move suddenly, or talk
in a loud voice. She
must listen, not inter-
rupt or contradict.
Her mother is tired
of her asking why.
She must not call attention
— like a stray dog —
to herself.
She must *pay* attention,
stand still, keep her
eyes on what moves,
be careful. Always
be careful. Because.

2

The girl must pay attention
to her mother, the traffic,
streetcar tracks, and old
people who get on the bus.
Let that lady sit down
her mother says, and
she does. The lady smiles,
says *thank you dear.*
Hang on! her mother says,
her voice a leash. *Stand*
still! She looks down
to the gleam of her patent leather
shoes. She will be careful
not to scuff them.

3

The girl must brush
her hair. She must
keep her eyes open and
her mouth shut.
She must watch her tongue.
She knows it means
'don't speak
to your mother
like that,' but wonders,
if she *could*
watch her tongue,
would it wag?
Would that mean
she was happy?

4

The girl must be polite
to everyone, even when
they interrupt her.
Put your book down!
her mother says. *Go*
outside, keep an eye
on your brother. There's
a good girl now. She will
pretend she is a sheep dog,
beautiful Lassie with
the flowing coat.
If she's careful she might
find her way home.

5

The girl must put things
away. She must pick up
after herself. Because.
Sniffing the yard one
whole afternoon,
digging out her brother's
lost toys, she puzzles
over how she might learn
to step along behind herself,
lean over, gather what
she has somehow already
dropped.

Friday Nights at 14

My games of cowboys and Indians forsaken,
the fields dissolved into streets where I trailed
girls with the right laughs and a certain cocky walk.

At the teen canteen my best friend and I danced.
Our circle skirts flew straight out
            our legs were strong and quick
                        we didn't miss a step.

Sometimes a boy noticed and asked me to dance,
folded his arms around my hunched shoulders
when the music slowed. I wanted
to burrow into him and never go home,
my nose hidden in his shirt,
his breath warm on the back of my neck.

Bye-bye Love

All that awkwardness and still I was sometimes
happy, laughing, singing *bye-bye love*
parading along the sidewalks after supper —
those long summer evenings
light stretching out a red-gold halo
over the rooftops and skittish cars
that paused
or honked and squealed away
bye-bye love trailing out the windows
down the street behind them.

A Moment's Absence

She imagines herself driving through countryside no longer familiar, the car seat soaking up the warmth of the sun and her leaning into it thinking *This is how it feels to be happy*, singing in spite of her tin ear and thin voice: *Remember the Red River Valley and the cowboy who loved you so true.*

In the back seat an album of pictures from last summer's vacation to show the great-aunt she imagines visiting, so the aunt will be able to see her life, full of husband and children, the things they have done.

She parks carefully beside the winter-bleached little house, the air surprisingly sweet, not the imagined rich manure smell of her childhood, but red clover and sweetgrass.

In the tiny living room scuffed linoleum, a tray with china teacups and silver spoons, her aunt pouring hot water into the teapot, and shortbread cookies out of a box with a plaid lid.

Sitting side by side on the chesterfield looking at the pictures, she imagines her aunt saying nothing as she turns the pages except to ask the names of the children or if she wants more tea. This looking takes a long time, the afternoon growing dim.

On the way home signs blur by, deepening twilight making it hard to see the road's edges clearly. Afternoon and road smudge sleepily together as she realizes she's not in any of the pictures. Or is she imagining this as well?

Turning from her desk, she sees the painting that hangs on the opposite wall. In it a wooden chair stands on a stone floor; from the floor's edge steps lead into space which is blue and pink; the room, if it is a room, is empty otherwise except for the shadow of a woman's body across the floor; the shadow's head falls outside the painting; her feet must be planted somewhere in the blue space.

Hating the Woman Next Door

1

Everything about her, lank hair,
hunched shoulders curved over her chest,
ragged hole of her mouth cursing
husband and children, invading
my workroom even through closed windows
on a Sunday morning. It could be
any morning, has been
almost every morning for months
since she moved in and turned
sullenly away from my forced
hello as I watched her, four children
clinging to her legs, struggling
up the front steps to her door.

I've pasted a black star map and
the poster of our blue planet
across my window that looks
into her kitchen: still
not enough distance between us.
She drives my daughters frantic.
They want to call the police, or anyone,
to shut her up, though they take
her side against her husband
while I'm ready to take up arms
with him, she our common curse. I'm
trying to write and she's shrieking *Shut*
your fucking mouth! for the third time
and goddamn bitch, I'm going to open
my window and scream back
If you're so fucking angry
do something about it! Leave!

But I'm above that here in my second floor
room and besides, I'm afraid of her,
believing the hunch in her shoulders might
explode, or worse, her voice name me
a reason for her sour rage.

I'd like nothing better
than to put us both
out of her misery.

2

It's years since I've thought of her,
but this morning I've remembered the dog,
a sleek red hound that howled constantly
from its chain in the backyard.
One afternoon it got away.
She stood on the front walk staring after it
as it tore up the street, silken-skinned,
gone with the wind.

"Beautiful dog," I said, and she nodded.
We stood there, the two of us, watching
the animal run.

What Happened

> ...it was running slowly, it ran for its life. Sometimes that can happen.
> JOHN BERGER, *and our faces my heart brief as photos*

I didn't know I had fallen asleep.
A voice echoed and echoed.
His hair was long and curling.
It was only a shape.
I wish to suggest nothing except it was time to leave.
A voice was going on and on.
I'd been waiting for years and my shoulders ached.
A black shape edged along the side of the bed.
A door must have been left open.
I suppose I'd always known he would come.
My daughter says *it's me it's me it's me*
He didn't go away.
I don't want to insist on anything.
She wants to throw up, her head is reverberating.
His hair lifted in dark flames above his head.
I must have had something on my mind.
I'm sitting up, I'm not dreaming.
A voice is going on and on.
Her head is pounding and it won't stop.
A dark shape flares at the top.
The thin sound won't stop.
She says her head hurts.
Someone is screaming.
A black shape stands there.
She's sick.
I suggest nothing, I insist on nothing.
She stands beside the bed.
I'm sitting up, I'm screaming.
She is not a dream.
A door was left open.
Sometimes that can happen.

This House Is Full of Longing

Even the walls grow dizzy with it, losing their focus,
dreaming themselves toward some less substantial form
the wind blows through. The doors wish themselves
music swinging on their hinges while the pictures
on the wall yearn toward some other dimension as we sit
wrapped in our own thoughts, evening curling round us.

What dimension might contain this moment nascent
with such longing, the child mounting the stairs,
the young woman poised at the doorway, each carried
by her own quickening hunger for the possibility
she may become? A tremor ripples out from this centre
disturbing the trees as the rain slicks the street,
shush, shush, and the house fills with the pulsing of wings.

Fear of Knives: the Prairie

Always there, the horizon line, always looming, the sky,
and windy silence so thick she could cut it with a knife,
herself spilling out unknowable distances, thinning,
thinning, till she snapped back into that other prospect,
the sharp edge of a blade raising a horizon line of blood
against the soft and subtle imaginings of skin,
anything at all wet and blooming welcome in this dry air,
the gurgle of life let out to feed the space and wind.

That's how it might have been looking out the farm door
across all those plants whose names she didn't know.
The shimmering miles of endless delicate repetition,
the children hanging for dear life onto her knees,
and her standing aproned and framed in the wooden doorway,
holding that life sharp in her unsound implausible hands.

This poem is based on a story Anne Szumigalski told me when I asked her what it had been like to move to the prairies after growing up in England. It is dedicated to her, with her permission.

I Dance Country

It's raining across the whole country, I bet, slicking these heaped
Shield rocks red under a white sky lowering in and past the wind-
shield wipers' slur the road's edge flung with wildflowers gleams
like somebody's just spatter-painted it red, yellow, and white.
In Manitoba the wheat's still green and if you look you'll see
the wind punching up clouds upon clouds over yellow-green waves
as rain blows in streaking the window.

Drive — I said,
I've got him and the rain on my mind like in any good country song,
imagining we're dancing, pulled in to the tavern with the jukebox
or maybe (it's Friday night) a three-piece Western band.
It's so real I can feel his arm across my back stronger than I
remembered it and dancing like this is all I ever want to do,
nothing's so perfect thirty years down the road as country music
and his arms, this riddling mix of memory and desire swinging me home.

The highway rises to meet wet cloud along the North Shore,
it's late afternoon and the road swoops like any crow in and out
of fog, the land looming up shadowy and blurred and any story
might be happening out there past the rocks and pines, the swamp
where moose browse like no one's ever stopped but only hightailed
past through the rain to the next jukebox and hot cup of coffee and
these wheels turning keep the dream alive, I'm still dancing.

It's getting dark now as we drive and the rain still falls. The road
reeks of emptiness, the land is only shadow, it's hard to see
anything but the road's sleek skin and rock and trees edging in.
There's no tavern round this curve and no jukebox, but the radio's on
to hurtin' songs and I want to look up and see myself glowing
in the blurry windshield, looking more beautiful than he ever
remembered me, his glance holding me here as we dance, buoyed by
the rain and the dark and the road, this country music leading us on.

Transactions

She's been thinking for hours about the man at the camera store,
all the conversations they've traded while film and pictures
changed hands. He comes from Saskatchewan.
Once she was wearing her straw hat and he reached out
and touched its brim as softly as if it were skin,
and she knew he thought she looked
wonderful and that left to its own accord his hand
would have brushed her cheek.
She was startled and stepped back.
He's younger than she is and prairie handsome and for a few days
afterwards she walked as if she wore a shawl of prairie sunshine
and was dazzling in it.

Yesterday going to the lakeshore with her daughter
she met him in the subway with his kids.
As they got off the train at the same station
they exchanged remarks and he put his hand gently to her back
shepherding her ahead of him and all evening as she listened
to country music and cleaned the closets she wondered
what it would be like to kiss him, imagining
his face bending toward hers.

All of Saskatchewan opened out behind him awash in sunlight,
its uncertain distance, and she knew her wish to be awash
in that distance again was at least half her wanting to kiss him.
That night she dreamed they holidayed at the same camp.
One misty afternoon she met him in a screened-in sleeping loft.
He wore white shirt and shorts and he smiled, opening his arms to her,
and kissed her with such tenderness she woke suddenly and

Here the horizon is always lost behind buildings
the trees lean in clouding the sky and what she wants
is someone to make love to her
through this night's rain who has nothing to prove,

his hands sure and tender on her body which is strong
and ready to be moved.

Now she worries she'll be awkward when she picks up her pictures
on Wednesday, half-convinced it's him she wants, her wrists
anxious, offering themselves, her eyes squinting against the light.

A Form of Falling

I want you to know I like this — conversation
roving across the yard, the moon rising suddenly
and you, slightly thickened into the present,
sitting across the table from me.

Thirty years ago I opened a door and
your blue-eyed radiance stopped me short.
Did you know I loved you? I never
dared say *touch me* believing you'd say *no*,

but for years I dreamed repeatedly I was
standing in front of you as your head
bent toward me. Our lips never met. What
would happen if I leaned toward you now?

It's funny, this week I've dreamed of you
twice. I'm walking with you at top speed
toward some unspecified destination through
fields, along city streets, up a shaded drive —

Why did you abandon me?

— and now here we sit, your sons and my daughters
the distances from which we speak to each other,
laughing, a little surprised (at least I am)
at this awkward pleasure of being together.

You look at me through glasses you didn't have
and I'm feeling a certain blurriness of vision
should be cherished, the way I find myself
now cherishing your fading hair. I want

to ask you what you saw in me, what you
wanted. *I'm leaning toward you in the dark.*

Do you know your voice telling me things
is exactly the way I remember it? And if my body

settling toward the softness of that voice
persists in dreaming still — *your lips, your hands,*
here, oh here — perhaps that is merely
(merely?) another form of remembering

that sometimes we don't ask enough, full of desire
and thinking ourselves visible by its brilliance alone,
that loss like birth pushes us again and again
toward some unknown and unsought country.

Cleaning Cupboards

I'm wearing the belt buckle you gave me like a talisman
but still I say "Don't touch me!" my body lax
and uneasy, intent on something I haven't recognized.
There is a pasture emptying my head, I'm falling through space,
and I haven't asked you if there's a difference between
departure and drowning. The life I made up is so solid.

I wish I could walk toward you with flames flaring
from my shoulders. I wish I were rising like the fish
in your dreams, from some green river, sequined, glittering,
as lissome as gleaming snakes among the leaning ferns.

There are nineteen glasses, two egg cups, two shot glasses,
a coffee mug and a small bin of measuring cups and spoons
on the shelf I've just cleaned and four more cupboards to go.
It's the end of August and the rain is falling at last
creeping up through the basement drain with its burden
of dirt and old leaves, teasing the laundry heaped on the floor.
All this cleaning and things still grow musty.

Once you said to me "If I left my wife now it would be
to live in a cave." Today I say "I can't do this!"
Am I speaking to you or the cupboards? I don't know what
I'm hunting for. I don't even know the life I'd make up
for myself if I could find the door out of this house.

Sometimes Things Pause

Sometimes things pause and give a great roar —

like now, trees bent nearly double and
sirens caromming against the wind while
I'm caught on my friend's steps. Thunder
explodes, the key's stuck, my glasses are weeping,
and the wind's so fierce now
it swallows the sirens. Try though I do
I can't open the door. At home
my daughter's asleep under the flimsy roof
of her third-floor room, not knowing
the radio's blared a tornado watch.
My study door will blow shut with a crash
knocking the quiet flying.

Will it wake my daughter, asleep in
her third-floor room? I can't open this door,
and there's no one to ask about it. A life
has to begin somewhere so why not
here and now?

"I want to imagine being in my element, she said"
— DAPHNE MARLATT

Underwater

Dream of the Empty Shore

I'm here and not here where dusk stretches
and flows along an empty beach that curves
the edge of a lake near clattering reeds.
Birch trees — thin spirits — glimmer
and dissolve as darkness rises from the ground
stretching in its turn till it stands and fills the sky.
A small night wind plucks my shirt,
a shudder ripples through the reeds and
laps against my feet. Sighs fall from water
and trees, I'm here and not here, floating
slightly above myself, my feet tethered
in cold mud. Clouds part and pass behind
the moon, dissipating sound. Here, not here,
I sway in the night's spangled air as

the drowned don't speak but gather,
bruised and disruptive.

Death of a Marlborough Man

In memoriam F.B., February 1992

How we are betrayed by our bodies (and betray them).
How seductively images engage us, hungry as we are.
Even you, with your easy stance, your brooding glances
cast out into that middle distance.
Such mastery, your cool courtesy, those stories
that never included me, such technicolour temptations!

When you spoke, your resonant voice retrieving dreams,
mesas and desert plains filled in behind you,
that spacious and difficult landscape a polished surface
reflecting whatever stories propelled you to the cliff's edge
to speak over the emptiness, your fingers yellowed
and ash on the sleeve of your buckskin-coloured jacket.

That horse you leaned against as you smoked and stared across
the rumpled much-photographed country
must have nickered suddenly, its ears twitching, catching you
unawares. It stamped its feet. It carried you away.

Hunger

In memory of my cousin, Robert Brannan

I remember: lichen on rock, smell of blueberries mixed
with juniper and pine, salt on my upper lip from
the cooking sun, sounds of our feet cracking
twigs, crunch of old leaves and I want you back
Bobby, dead fifteen years in a lake, the plane
you were learning to fly crashed by your teacher.
I heard about it on the radio.

You've left me wailing in the bush, abandoned,
my fingers purple as my mouth, afraid of the bears
you pretended to hear, pawing toward me. I'm starving
in spite of the blueberries, and for years now
I've gnawed on the thin bone of a dream

that it was a mistake, the radio report,
that it wasn't you,
that I hadn't heard it in the half-light of not yet
having woken on a Sunday morning,
that there was no phone call later from my sister
telling me you were dead,
that I didn't stumble down the hallway refusing
to believe I was awake.

I want you back, Bobby, in spite of your
faithlessness, this shabby contrivance with
coincidence and a minor mishap on
the news. I want to scuff along
the sand of Pelican Lake behind you,
my feet warm, listening to you tell your friends
about the Americans who buy your minnows
for bait. I want to finish filling my basket with
blueberries while you wait. I want to come into
the crowded low-ceilinged kitchen for breakfast and
eat my fill
of the pickerel you've caught
amazed at what you've done while I was still asleep.

"Everything Is Changed"

In memory of Shirley Ann Wood (Jan. 28, 1934–Dec. 4, 1992)

1. December 1991: Waiting for Diagnosis

I think my sister-in-law is imagining herself dead.
The constriction in my throat is the grief of failure, my
helplessness, feeling her absence from her daughters' lives,
from her own, the emptiness she will leave.
Abandoned, abandoning, perhaps she feels herself derelict.

Severed from what she knows, she shrinks from every
glance. Her hand rises to her ruddy cheek, its slight
apple swelling that mimics health, that old woman
from fairy tales whose riddle contains
the solution to the problem.

One solution may
dissolve her, dissolving the suspended life
lying in wait. That one will carry her further out
along the swinging bridge over the gorge
whose purpose it is to separate her from
herself immersed in the familiar, embodied.

I see her hands clench as she sits curled at the end
of the bed. We are half-watching the television, half-
waiting for the messenger, any messenger,
who may say the word to unriddle this.

2. November 1992: Making Advent Wreathes

This morning the world wakes up white, its new thin skin
so pallid and delicate emerging suddenly from the dark
and the chairs I forgot to wash and bring in are oddly
at home, their yearning white arms and seats presenting
a different angle of expanse from the sloped white roofs
falling out of the blank white sky. The table is littered
with balsam boughs so dark they're almost black. It's still
cold and she's dying and

I'm thinking about winter, how
it will curve toward spring and this year the whole world
seems to be waiting. I imagine myself crouched
at the foot of a tree in the smoke-shrouded rain forest,
or at the edge of an iced and suds-filled river, or there,
in that hospital room. While the days labour like her
labouring to die, the earth grates on its axis, snow silts up
the windows, and day after day the grey ash sky blurs my eyes.

I'm waiting for her to be gone.

I want it over now, not blurred by this seasonal circling, this
ceremony of the dark and snow which says trust, soon
the earth will be bright again. Its brightness won't bring her.

It's her death, her particular difficult death, that I want
not to notice, as I wait for it, weaving balsam into the frames,
buying the red candles.

3. Snow Fell as Predicted

The dark comes so suddenly some nights.
The kitchen is cold. I've looked up
from the bright page and it's black
outside, even the lights next door are out,
and what I thought a star leaning in

is only a plane winking and passing.
I'm trying not to think about you.

The night before you died I dreamed
strange robotic monsters (matte-
finished, slightly sexual) lurked
near the elevator, the stairwell.
But we made our way out anyway to
the parking lot where the school bus waited
to take us on the excursion. We'd waited
a long time for this day.

Whatever waiting I'd been doing seemed not
nearly long enough, when the phone rang with the news.
Everything unspoken rings in my ears, not the words
I might have said to you, not those, you knew I loved you,
but the words of my own grieving, the way I
feel now, partial, aching, depleted.

4. October 27, 1993: The Legacy

You've been dead nearly a year now and I've
kept my back turned, not asked you in. I use the glass
salad bowls you gave me, thinking how much I like them,
but don't ask how you are or say I'm sorry,
I miss you. I do miss you, but I'm afraid of your gaze,
knowing how I stayed away from you at the end, crying
in my study, brushing up dried leaves from the plants.

I wish you were here. I want to tell you how
empty my house seems some days. You know, it's not
that being-good life we talked about I want
for myself any more. I think about the tears we shared,
hanging onto each other hard, while we still
believed there was more than one answer to the riddle.

lost children

still and noiseless, eyes closed, curled in upon
himself, his feet have shrivelled, those
long skinny legs have webbed together, calcium
threads binding him beneath a sea where
he is held, laved in salt

swaddled in silence my lost son lies
in my throat, dried leaf, antique snail, curled
at the base of my tongue, swallowing my words

salt crust in my throat, my mouth gritty as sand
I can't remember his cry

**

I'm twenty-one years old (in the basement) crying.
I'm twenty-five years old (in the library) crying.
I'm twenty-nine years old (holding my daughter) crying.
I'm thirty-five years old (with fragments of poems) crying.
I'm thirty-seven years old (pregnant) crying.
I'm forty-three years old (walking to work) crying.
I'm fifty years old (holding my book of poems) crying.

**

across the room   they held him up some distance
away   I suppose so I couldn't reach for him or
touch him   red scrap with my face

A Walk by the Dugout

Any place on the circumference is
an entrance. The field behind
the dugout, for instance.

In the field the flowers are
riotous, a toss and tangle, a fling
of scent poured out by the sun's
heated touch.

Above the field three crows
raucous a hawk, banging, clanging,
their black calls relentless
teetering its steady flight.

But turn from digression, even
from the world's sweet presence and
ask your hard question.
What remains?

What remains but the hard
block in my chest my hands full
of breaking and my own
loneliness?

Mudra: the Empty Bowl

1

Water is inexhaustible. It streams out of the downpipes on the sheds in gushes. The thundering grey sky pours down.

The day after the day I dreamed I was drowning, I walked around the dugout attended by a cloud of blue dragonflies stitching through the swaying brome. I found three magpie feathers, one which was standing up in a clump of grass beckoning to me. Everything shone.

My eyes too. So much shining.

2

Here at the edge of the dugout the trees fall away and the distance stands up around me. The line of spruce bordering the road throws its image upside-down into the water. Slightly dizzy, I face that doubling in the fading light of a cloudy evening. So still.

Beyond the water, beyond the spruce trees, boundless sky and empty fields blend. Everything comes to this — a pause where the material world thins and questions.

Light, air, distance and longing, the mirror water. Waiting.

3

Days and days of no messages. The owl drifting up from the creek last night meant nothing, it disappeared back along the meadow. The trees are empty. My mouth is dry. In the bush where I sit under a spruce, a few feathers scattered and the dead wing of a thing. Old leaves. I will sit here and let my skin fall into the ground, become bark, pebbles, dirt.

4

Forgive me, I have not thrived. I have lived without abandon, my feet heavy in the ground. I have practiced goodness and fallen short believing I knew, even in the cacophony of voice and argument, of necessary and needless pain. I have floated rootless and drowning, held my tongue, denied the flood. I have not cried beside the river. I have failed to stand up in the light and the dark. Forgive me.

I have not thrived.

failure to thrive

she thinks it will never end or end too quickly
this short summer before they move, leaving
behind this house where she doesn't feel at home
now, where everything familiar pushes against
her, even her own body, its unusual roundness,
its unpleasant and vivid smells, its distant
detachment, as if it no longer housed her

she wants to refuse that body, slide out of it,
abandon its leaky messes, its pure hollowness
where once life was rumoured, she wants it
to get thin, fall away to its bones,
and the bones to grow translucent,
letting the summer sun shine through, licking
them clean
                                        she stares through the screen
door waiting to disappear into whatever
is out there, feel of morning on her bare
arms, articulate and harsh longing, thin skin

she dreams the cells of her body licked up
by the wind, herself diaphanous, insensible, absorbed
into that field, its trodden grass
paths, tangle of clover and foxtails, stones
by the creek, anything but this thick-
tongued, stupid, unhearing, awkward, empty body

Clear Light

Morning is the moment when the light shifts, its tone now a sure memory of blue instead of the blurred grey or sepia from a moment ago. "The clear light of a new day" we say and I see what we mean. The cedar stands out against the snow where once it flattened into it.

Today I didn't see that blue arrival. My gaze had fallen from the brown blur beyond the window to my hands settled in my lap and then I had remembered Kathie. Bleakness rose over me like a beam of light scrubbing away the traces of who I was when her eyes were on me.

I'm trying to tell you about the face that lies beneath the face, the one that rises to the surface from time to time, summoned by someone who recognizes it even before it looks up.

When I looked at the trees again they were sharp-edged and the light was sharp too. I'd only glanced away for an instant, a second at most, but that was long enough to miss the shift from blur to blue. One time I saw a sky the palest of greens before the sun broke through. I tried to photograph it but the colour didn't hold.

The mind falls so fast.
Kathie's been dead six months now.
Who am I when the light shifts?

Blue Willow

All the summer houses lie in the east, another
country, they rise from the vertical plates, the round bowls
in the cupboard. I sit and watch them through the glass.
Someone stands on a bridge, she is slender, her head
is bent, her hand lies on the railing.
I try it myself on the porch, but no river runs away
from beneath my feet. I can imagine the music
as the willows sway, as the woman sways, walking.
To walk across China to the pavilion.

She will step off the bridge on the other side of the river
and disappear along the path behind the willows
into her unwatched life, which I think must be
an invisible and melancholy story of a broken heart,
the man she loves not noticing the grace of her silent walk.
The way she stands watching the water
means sadness.

At thirteen I already believed in broken hearts as the higher story.
I believed in the fine thinness of blue willow china
letting the light through, the unutterable beauty
of what might shatter if touched. I trusted the delicacy
of the bent head.

What I am asking for now is not so much —
only the footbridge arcing from beside the willows across
the water, and someone murmuring a shy song.
To walk across China to the pavilion holding your hand.
To find in a summer house a blue bowl of nasturtiums,
these friends, wholehearted conversation, and the way
the music washes over us, lifting us up.

River Mud

Did he fish? Hunt for frogs? Cut willow sticks for arrows and spears? Did he roll down the bank, over and over under the sun? She thought the boy must have insisted on playing on the riverbank the way she had herself, but she couldn't really imagine *him*, only a boy's life such as she herself might have led, had tried to lead when she was ten, dreaming of riding buckskin horses at high speed for the pony express, delivering the message that would avert disaster *just* in the nick of time.

She imagined there was, however, a difference between them. He went in and out of the river, absorbed but careful, unafraid. Unlike her who thought endlessly about falling and typhoid and being swept away by the silky brown water.

Along the riverbank, she remembered, it was always mud at the water's edge. Not sand. Sand belonged to lakes. The river owned mud, wiping and polishing, making it smooth and shiny as black silk. When it left off its polishing and withdrew for a rest, the sun slowly sucked away the dark smoothness which, going, left deep fissures in its place, odd shapes with edges that curled up slightly, hinting at enigmatic patterns.

She remembered the peculiar smell of mud at the river's edge, musty, a little sour, green. She wondered if that was the taste in his mouth as he drowned, the taste in hers now as she remembered.

What Can I Make from My Sadness?

A greyish-brown spider crawls up the spines of the books piled on my study floor. I watch it for a moment, then put a glass over it. Now I don't know what to do. I wonder if it's a jumping spider. Tiny black and white ones live in my study. They leap like frogs along the windowsill when I put my giant finger near.

Kathie liked spiders. Or at least she made room for those she found in her house. She spoke of reading their webs for a sense of direction and even, with apology, removed the one that lived behind her toilet tank when the plumber was coming. I think she put it in her bedroom.

When I came back from my summer holidays I gave her a photograph which she pasted on the wall by her bed. She was dying then. I'd taken the picture when I went deep-sea fishing, out from P.E.I. into the evening ocean, a place Kathie knew. On the trip back to shore we seemed to journey inside a shell, ocean and sky alike gone opalescent as the sun went under cloud and sank to nightfall. I was full of euphoria, surrounded by mother- of-pearl. All I could think was *Why is there something instead of nothing?* I could hear no sound above the wind's sound. Its deep cool brushed my arms.

I've had the spider under a glass for three days now. The glass is cold when I touch it and the spider just sits. I still don't know what to do. Outside it's raining but there's snow and ice on the ground. The wind huffs up. Three days and I don't know if it has moved. This morning I dreamed the glass was empty. The question I was supposed to ask was *Why is there nothing instead of something?*

"within the bound world of the disconsolate"

a found poem for my unnamed stillborn brother*

too slight, too ephemeral to merit attention ...
the tiny bones of babies —
often buried at birth ... in Languedoc ...
have been discovered —
... rejected —
buried beneath the mud floors of protohistoric dwellings ...
[in Languedoc]

each minuscule collarbone
each shoulder blade
(no wider, often, than a periwinkle)
the seedling of each incisor still locked
within the slender husk of its jawbone ...
sole remaining vestige ...

the fetus, the stillborn, and the dead nursling ...
so tenuous ...
in a wrapped fetal position,
their knees brought level with their chin ...
their spinal columns ... a near self-enveloping ellipse ...

cheek of one stillborn baby ...
discovered lying against a tiny collection of pebbles ...
of another cradled in the minuscule cup
of one of its hands ...

absolutely nothing distinguishes this soil
[in Languedoc]

these infant deaths ...
their tiny bodies ...
with little or no ritual ...

abandoned
— flung —
to the elements themselves ...

flexed little corpses —
often not much larger than a rabbit ...
inscribed within vestige itself ...

withheld ...
[in Languedoc]

those who'd never (or scarcely)
even existed ...
'here' ...
within the bound world of the disconsolate ...

**from Gustaf Sobin, "Baby Burials: Domestic Inhumation in the Iron Age" in* Luminous Debris.

Threnody: Reasons for Mourning Ken Saro-Wiwa

Because I didn't think it would happen.
Because the sun streamed undisturbed into my kitchen when the radio announced his hanging.
Because I didn't believe what I heard.
Because I knew him only as an empty chair in a tumult of language, a possibility.
Because that possibility was violence and I had believed in the equal possibility of rescue.
Because I hadn't read his books.
Because he had several children and was sometimes Anglican.
Because this November was only rain and heavy grey skies, then snow.
Because complacency is within reach and familiar.
Because I didn't know the names of the others.
Because I think he was a good enough man and it wasn't enough.
Because some of us are pleased he is dead.
Because I'm afraid.
Because the skies darken and darken over flaring oil wells and we look away.
Because there are people cradling a leg or an arm, all that remains of someone they loved.
Because his mother was horsewhipped in the course of his trial.
Because the trial was a farce.
Because I wonder if he felt he had nothing to lose.
Because they had to try five times to hang him.
Because his marriage failed and he gave up his publishing business to take to the streets with the Ogoni.
Because the Ogoni are dying and may disappear.
Because I might not have liked him.
Because it's the turn of the year and I can't tell if it turns up or down.
Because I'm fifty-two years old and only beginning to know what I want.
Because he died at fifty-four.
Because I'm afraid of the dark and smoke-filled countryside.

Because the Malawi poet Felix Mnthali wrote that he went to his death
singing, they all went to their deaths singing.
Because I can't carry a tune.

Toronto, November 1995

This poem is written against forgetting:
Baribor Bera, Saturday Dobee, Nordu Eawo,
Daniel Gbokoo, Dr. Barinem Kiobel,
John Kpuinen, Feliz Nuate, Chief Rewane,
Ken Saro-Wiwa.

Be the River

Be the river then, straight or crooked,
its hidden energy pulling it ever *down*
at a speed that's barely visible. Be
its red clay trough, be the way it wears
its own being-in-motion into place there,
the polished and runnelled banks which
curve and hold, be both flow and bank
and then the rising above. Be the air above
which pushes against its surface smoothing
or ruffling, snatching for something.
Be the tangle of small willows crowding
the bank, leaning over their reflections,
growing dizzy watching the clouds drift
among the fish beneath them. Be willows
and be too the stones in the gravel bank
whose slight movements mirror the way
water meets air, who bask in weather
and are patient. Be the silt washing in
from the rain, and the muskrat swirling
at the bank, be the splash and trickle of
sounds without identity, half-formed words
surfacing, do you hear? Be the swallows
who skim along the water's surface twisting
their narrow wings to rise and dart and
dip down again. Be all these and more,
whatever falls into the water and through
its skin to find the robust and hidden depths,
tumbling towards its wide mouth, singing.

We Weave Our Lives from Grief and Call It Other Things

One winter solstice we punched holes in all
the tin cans from the blue box and stuck
candle stubs in them and set them fluttering
on the snowy lawn. It was cold, I don't
remember if there were stars, and my 12-year-old
daughter and her three friends stamped about
following her father and chanted over their lanterns
Go away dark, come back light
while the two 20-year-olds thought whatever
they thought, their faces wavering above
the candle flames, their tin lanterns
held, contemplated, set down in the snow.

I don't know what all this has to do with grief
exactly, but it's come to mind as I think of
my friend's grief workshop, and what
does it means to be practised, at ease
with the squirrel squashed in the street,
the one-footed pigeon at the bus stop,
or my sister-in-law's dying?

I want to say time passes or things change
as if these notions were a kind of answer, but
who asked what question? Grief trails through
our lives like Chinese lanterns hung in a garden,
not paper but tin like the ones we set down
in the snow, glittering, reflective, making
holes in the dark. I see how we are summed up
in the light of these lanterns as if
we were the flames, illuminating ourselves,
dreaming we can reach out for an instant
and touch, making our own light in the dark.

Sleepless

Mind racing, legs twitching. Sleep a continent away. Held by the half-dark she aches to move. *Do something!*

Slide out of bed, stand under the revolving fan. Air pushes across her neck, down her body. Something subsides and settles. She wants to move and disturb nothing.

She sees herself glide, a shadow, down the stairs. To the window over the sink. The moon hangs in the branches of the oak tree. She stands under the fan and sees herself there, almost transparent.

Pick up a book and carry it to the yard. Watch the moon slide through the leafy branches. Listen — to whatever sounds linger in the not-deep darkness — small swish of traffic from the main street two blocks away — a bird's startled call — leaves and plants rustling in the wind —

Oh, the wind! It moves like air from the fan. She wants to stand beneath the heavy canopy of the oak and feel it against her arms. She wants to sleep. She can't. *Is this what it all comes to?* Standing under the fan she feels the half-dark pressing iron plates against her chest. She wants to push back. She can't. When she tries, her hands go right through.

December, Reading the Sky

Light fails, night falls, my heart too —
What became of this day?

It began well — sky flushed rose
Behind drifts of charcoal clouds
And light floating off to either side
Offering December's clear promise.

O I love the north at this time of year,
Its incomparable high skies.

Mid-morning, puzzling over
The pigeons' repetitive calligraphy,
I saw a hawk — exclamation mark —
Perched on the antenna below them
Deciphering their flight. Neither
Of us moved for some time and
Nothing further happened.

What should have happened?

Now it's evening, sky darkening. Why
Is there never anyone home when
You want them? My mother
Hasn't called me once since she died.

I Must Change My Life: Homage to Rilke

I look up and I look up.
Each time you enter the room.
It's these long twilights, the kind we had at home across
that field behind the house by the railway tracks where
the clouds flew up at evening.
These books, this music, my life — how could
I have forgotten?

I'm trying to surrender despair, that
helplessness.
I'm trying to walk under this umbrella, love, its
stiff jointed arms, its silken
fabric, its awkward angling
embrace.
I look up and it's surrounded by sky.

I've entered the room where the drapes are blowing,
the floor gleams, the furniture is quiet.
This canopy, that desk with the flowers,
my jointed arm stiff from writing.
I look up and I look up and —

Each time it's you entering the room,
surrounded by sky.

My hands are full of words in
the evening distance, space
where wind combs the field at twilight, clouds
flying up.

I wanted to drag a few words out of silence then sleep and none
were what I truly wanted. So much silence and so many words.
— JIM HARRISON, "Ghazal LVII"

How Do I Know My Name?
Ghazals

Ghazal 1

for John Thompson

How do you write a poem? How do I know my name?
The cat's got my tongue, who stole my words?

I have no son, I have no lover.
And now I have no husband.

Let me now (not) to the marriage of true words
admit impediment. My feet are granite and ivory.

It's the firmament on which we stand and
which soars above us, the great surround.

Everywhere is the centre of the world
said Black Elk.

Brought to my knees, helpless, who I am,
my voice the one I speak in.

Bulletins from the Inner World (Ghazal 2)

There are papers everywhere, buried wings.
The noise is deafening.

Each morning we've woken to rain.
Trees are staggering, tulips drunk.

Some days there's no place to sit
beneath an opalescent sky.

The tire track on the verge tells me nothing.
All the things that speak, you too, are unhelpful.

This closet, this box of books, this room.
My occupation, my leaning, my falling down.

Menopause Ghazal

Menopause —
It's no pause, it's my life!

At this exact moment the bells ring out
and it's lunchtime.

O language, you faithless lover,
fleeing my languid glance.

What's left, what's left over —
Who can tell the difference.

Ah restlessness, you make the days
hang together.

Ghazal 3: Name Games at St. Peter's

The intoxication of naming: western red lily, merlin,
musquash *(Ondatra zibethica)*, sweet red raspberry.

Thomas, Basil, Demetrius, Gerald, Anthony, Peter.
Lorna, Barbara, Jane, Joanne, Carol, Catherine, Liz.

Simon says, *I have never, no never ...*
What belongs and what doesn't is a constant worry.

The subject of the traditional ghazal was usually love.
Warthog, Grasshopper, Traditional — then there's gin.

The clandestine order of words and laughter.
In the rough circle do we choose or find our places?

Ghazal 4: For the Clover-Strewn Verge

Attend to sadness, Rilke said, *be alone.*
Receive the future and your fate will emerge.

The approaching dust could be anybody's dark lover.
I sit by the roadside and watch the distance.

Your drunken, amatory tongue is thick with history.
The song says things come together then they come apart.

This beloved who limps is surely not the wanted one.
On the desk: crow feather, pinecone, a field stone.

I want, I want —
Some shadowy thing raises its head, stretches, leans forward.

By Any Name: Ghazals 5 and 6

When someone knocks at the door, think that he's about
To give you something large: tell you you're forgiven ...
ROBERT BLY, "Things to Think"

To speak directly would be a new thing.
It's sadness again, wearing the same old trope.

If I imagine largeness at the door, Robert,
I might not answer its knock. That's my same old voice.

Each day after each meal I walk around the dugout.
I'm after the dizzying fall into reflection.

A simple sentence consists of subject, verb, complement.
I love Saskatchewan, or, *My son is alive.*

In the end we agree English syntax lacks regimentation.
I don't even know his name.

**

My son is alive and his name is Stuart.
With a thin wail Sean gives up the ghost.

Twice-born, twice-stolen. Memory's a liar.
It licks up the dish of milk and leaves nothing.

Walking near the orchard in the late afternoon
I hear an owl calling *Who? Who?*

In all the fairy tales the prince is named Charming
and the changeling is named Changeling.

Names are tangled in my throat. How can nothing
have so many shapes and be so hard to hang onto?

Ghazal for my 57th Birthday (7)

I'm tired of speaking backwards,
the past in my throat.

The late train that no longer runs,
yet people wait on the platform.

The mouse runs up the clock
and light falls along the hall.

Was there anyone there to talk to?
The backyard is empty of all but dry leaves.

At the head of the stairs, a shadow.
The old sorrows, were they, too, late?

What I mean *is*

Bull's Head Ghazal

Open the book with a bull's head and the moon on its cover
but be careful what you summon.

I could use a little comfort, a little rest,
a sigh, an easy song.

Small cries drift from the conifers,
words in the language of crossbill.

In dream after dream we pull
against each other. He wins.

The grit of sleeplessness and sorrow
is hard as dust on the eyes.

Ghazal 8: Sleep

O sleep sleep sleep, why do you abandon me?
I lie tossed up like sea-wrack on a scratchy beach.

Words, nothing but words, wherever I turn, going
in and out the windows, in and out the windows.

The soiled skin of things veils the moon and
clouds my thoughts. Its transparency alters everything.

The sigh of the heater, the sigh of the wind
and the sigh of my own breathing.

That four-legged fellow running at night,
he's hunting and singing — *exemplum.*

Ghazal 9: Winter

Snow dances towards my window like it did for Kay and Gerda.
In my mind a door has opened and there you stand.

A cardinal breaks ice from a cedar bough.
She sits outside the window with it gleaming in her beak.

Is it you by Forgetful River, begging for spare change?
I have a handful of shredded Kleenex and broken peanuts for the birds.

We forget some things, lose some, throw some away,
like the shards of ice and mirror flung by the storm.

Oh, the past never gets older.
As if it were only yesterday it throws itself at your feet.

Rock Ghazal

Drink deep drink deep the poet sings.
What's a life without anguish and pretense?

When my mother arrived at Union Station
I could see she wasn't sure who I was.

Passion begins in the garden.
It ends at the tomb.

I come back to my room
but nothing has changed since I left.

My own petrified heart.
O rock, you're a hard place.

Ghazal 10: A Door Is Ajar

There's been a gate in my mind for days.
Some words stick in my throat, some I spit out.

The thirteenth day and still I know nothing.
The field where the corn grew is only half-planted.

This morning five crows croak from the elms.
And yes, by the dugout, the muskrat glances at me again.

Abbott Jerome has mowed the grass paths in the bush.
Bruno and Osualdus are pushing up daisies.

Everything belongs.
Nothing must be   can be   *is*   left out.

A door is ajar.
The gate, the gate is a gape

The Last Day

Wring it out, your old fantasy — the one
where you both stay and disappear.

Tuft of deer's hair in the electric fence and
a path that runs out before reaching the edge of the field.

At the long and blurred horizon — silence, whiteness, fog.
What is this longing for erasure?

In all this space is there a word waiting to break loose?

The spruce cone has opened on the desk
offering its deeds to the wooden surface.

Everything that drowns returns to us as cargo.
— ESTA SPALDING, "the anatomy of freighters"

The Drowned Boy

1. The Drowned Boy

Somewhere a boy is drowning. Or has drowned.
But he doesn't know it. He believes he is still
holding his mother's hand, still stepping carefully
along the dock's edge astonished by the sunset sky.
His face is lifted to the heavy light, the way
it trembles and darts through the gentle water.
Does his mother dream she flings him from her
in an agony because a bee plunges and stings her?
Its venom whorls below her skin, voices
keening at the membrane behind her ear, the thin-
bladed whine more than she can bear. *It all
happened so fast.* That's why he hasn't noticed
that his eyes blink slowly against water not light.
Ribbon weeds caress him soft as a mother's hand
and he yawns and drifts slightly, it's that dreamy
time of evening when some people leave
their bodies seated in padded green armchairs
while they spiral like augers through the dusk.
They believe they may glimpse the faces they had
before they were born — or at least the faces
of the mothers they never knew. As for
the drowned or drowning boy, a length of something —
weed, rope, plastic pipe — has caught him
under one arm. Perhaps it is this line he mistakes
for his mother's hand. Sometimes on a standstill night
when the moon is brightening, if you look closely
you'll catch sight of him, turning and shifting in the water.
You might see his eyes refract the light and flash
it back to yours, a blessing passing between.

2. Drifts Closer

Tonight his face is a scream —
train whistle shriek —
whatever you've dreamed of privation and confinement.
His eyes have rolled back in his head,
the fronds of his hair lift and his wet face
is wetter than before, smooth weeping wet,
his round O mouth hollow and soundless.
Something three fields away cries *Mother!*
across the tree roots, below the twittering
leaves, as the night stars wheel down
— it is always *down* — to the horizon. His hair fronds
lift and lift but he does not, *will not*,
rise from the water and walk. His head
is empty, his hand empty, there is nothing
to hold, no one whose fingers grasp his, only
this eddying bump and drift, this
aimless ease. All the passing night
he longs and longs and longs.

3. Misses His Mother

Empty-handed under the dock, alone,
his eyes wet. Somewhere in the world he imagines
his mother is crying. She wanders across fields, her sweater
torn, twigs in her hair, with her poor mismatched shoes
stumbling her feet on the furrows.

It *must* be like that, somewhere — a woman
in black, black hair matted, crying and
calling with a ripped and fading voice, her
eyes red and sore. The dust thrown up.

There's so much dust in the air. She can't
have forgotten him, can't have gone on
without him, leaving him to this murky light,
the muddy path through the trees that leads
only to the dock with its thin, frangible edge.

4. Imagines His Boyhood

He plays hockey on the river ice,
the frozen roads. He wraps magazines
over his shins, dons his mitts
and leans low over the curved stick.
He wants to slide across the rutted ice
but his wet feet stutter, begin to stick.
He falls and struggles up.

His mother takes him to the dump
looking for bottles and he finds shotgun
shells. They go to a movie in the heat
of August, wrapping the cool dark
around them. He sits silent inside
the soundtrack drinking coke.
He wipes his mouth with his hand,
wet fingers salty from the popcorn.

He gets a job after school delivering
groceries in the heavy basket of his bike.
The pedals balk, the bike skids and
he has to push it uphill. He plays
baseball till twilight blurs the lines,
hearing the wind ruffle the creek
while he waits to steal home.

5. Grows Up

The boy drifts through the flooded basement to the stairs,
rises above the water and ascends to the rooms where
there are tables and chairs, a cupboard with a vase
in it, his scribbler, a hockey stick and
the scuffed silence he almost hears,
light falling into the empty room where
his mother sits and sits, where he doesn't fit,
his voice bruising the silence, making her cry. His feet
on the floor are revolvers, are clattering
accusations, raucous black crows, mocking mocking —

When he grows up he'll build a dance hall with rainbow lights
strung round it and music thick with trombones.
The men's arms will scissor back and forth in red jackets making
sound ripple out and he will drift and sway
on its currents, twirling round, his feet like
feathers, like floating reeds, like blackbirds over
the dry fields of October darting, gathering, circling —
a whole flock of them together.

6. Goes for a Walk

The drowned boy has come out of the water.
Out for a stroll with his hair eddying
around him he feels at home in the dull rain.
He tastes the watery air and smiles. Cloud,
field, all the dull bronzed world has gone soft,
its edges blurred. Sounds travel a long distance
under the wet sky and bump up against
his brooding. He is not bothered by them,
does not really listen: tractor, magpie,
the rattling corn, this hum trailing past him
carried off in his wake. He doesn't bother
to look either, drifting along the grassy paths —
all that washed hair flung out for the rain to rinse.
Fields spin through his floating thoughts. Clouds
of dragonflies spiralling in the dusk. The wind's current
parting the grass makes a dance step seize
his ankles so he pirouettes, tossing his head,
shaking out his coloured thoughts
as a ruffed grouse ripples and expands
at the edge of the woods.

7. Meets the Drowned Girl in the Hall of Reeds

A fateful but accidental meeting, completely random. The slightest shift in a current would have changed everything, sweeping the drowned boy past the grasping reeds. If the wind had come up or the rain down he would not have floated there to amble through these stately weeds, abstracted and drifting from thought to thought, fingers trailing behind like memory —

— finding himself face to face with the drowned girl held fast among the watery grasses, their grasp wound around her ankles and calves, curling about her arms, holding her tightly to themselves. His fingers flowed across her face.

Hero and heroine, prince and princess, all those drowning stories played their parts in the wind which sprang up only to meander. There was no tower, no fearful forest, just a dreamy night and the rain of stars, an afterimage of light washing across the sky.

8. Finds a Boat on the Lake Bottom

Tripped on his morning amble toward a shore
he catches himself, drifts upright and
stares at peeling boards and rusted oarlock,
his pliable fingers kneading the punky wood
protruding from the lake's bottom,
half-bandaged with roots and weeds, critters
runnelling their lives within it,
held fast.

The boy remembers how the wind shakes
the lake's surface as a boat drifts and
hours trail toward evening.
Does he see
a man walking along a dock,
tackle box and pole in one hand?
The man's heart is a knot
pulled tight, so tight it stops
at the lake's edge and gives in,
held fast.

Waterlogged, the drowned boy twists and
turns away, his own heart
knotting. Something is flying
behind him, its shadow
rippling along the lake's surface.
That wind, hunting
him, osprey eyes glinting.
He can't catch his breath,
held fast.

9. Half Wakes Remembering

Another life, he can almost hear it. Not
his mother's voice calling but a kind of clear
hard music drifting through bright rooms,
tall pillars, low treed hills behind him.

A place of angels dancing, their feet brisk
as hummingbirds. His feet are uncertain on
the high and difficult steps, he doesn't know
where they lead, the room he was meant to go to.

The sky has lowered over the lake and snow
is threatening. If only he could remember —
a sound of bells at the end of the hall, and then —
He was there once when voices sang the evening forward,

people leaning in their chairs to listen as
the gentle hills moved closer. His body was left behind,
he had no hands and didn't need them. His shoes
were soft red leather and made no sound as he danced.

10. Goes Dancing with the Drowned Girl Beneath the Stars

At the moment the waning moon broke free of a cloud they turned to each other, heads bowed slightly, adrift in a grassy meadow. Their hands joined and they began a slow swirl, a slight dance that rocked against the nodding trees.

Her hair floated out on the night air, shiny beneath the moon, while his eyes winked and shone mimicking the dancehall's rainbow lights. The wind's music turned them, linked their hands, bumped shoulders and knees, tangled then freed them from the grass.

Through the whole evening they bobbed their heads like dandelions on a summer day when the wind never stops blowing and the clouds never stop scudding. Blow and blow till the seeds tear off and fly away.

At some moment her ankle catches on a root and his hand slips away from hers, his eyes blank in the bubbling air, the moon retires, and off he drifts. The stars were still above her, the night sky aglitter, a heavenly dome flung over and full of winking lights, strings of them falling down like dust.

11. On the Day of the Dead

On the Day of the Dead the drowned boy rises early,
packs his lunch and sheds his flesh for the walk
to the graveyard. His bony feet clack along the shore
and over the pebbles, his mad grin courts the sky
and the trees' cloak ripples out behind him.
Oh the wind's dance is mournful and gay, is *triste*,
is whispered music nibbling at his jaw, the whorl
of his ear and he hums back to it, hmmmm, hmmmm.

His handful of marigolds droops and the sugar cone
melts, sticky among his fingers, but still he grins,
imagining the party, its gossip and laughter, sound
of his mother's fingers on piano keys, his father
filling a glass, clattering spoons, and the way twinkling
lights revolve as his feet circle the dance floor.
Someone with long hair leans toward him, smiling,
hand held out, or so it seems, as a whisper draws him
outside to the field, the wavering trees, and
the sound of faint singing sliding into the lake.

12. Dreams of Speaking

Oh, Oh, Oh, he cries, the round O bubbles rising
into the empty air as he turns in his sleep
over and over again as easy as fish,
as birds circling above the lake.
His eyes are shut, his mouth opens and closes
like a nestling's, he wants to spit out
something: seeds or sounds.
He dreams a music of words humming
through the muffled wash here where he's rocked to sleep,
words sinuous and extravagant, murmuring closer.
They are dredging a track for him beneath
the clouded moon, out into a mown field
where someone is waiting —
his mother in black, the girl he danced with,
a great bird he once saw skimming the lake,
its wings just above the water

13. Metamorphosis

Say the Drowned Boy was washed free of the reeds and mud,
past the docks and bobbing boats, the drowned pines, past
the marsh with its cattails and red-winged blackbirds calling,
and was flung full-length on the beach, half in, half out of the water.

Say he lay face up on the muddy sand
the muskrats tunnelling around and under him.
Say there were snow geese and sandhill cranes
falling stars and northern lights
as the moon leaned forward across the sky.

The sun shone and shone on the glittering shore the day
a child stumbled over him, or a girl stopped at his feet.
Say he opened his eyes then, stared at the blue sky, felt
the scritch of sand on his bare shoulders, and decided
to stand. *You're it!* someone said, tagging his elbow.
Say he chased her beach after beach, laughing,
breathing, gasping, no longer drowning.

NOTES

When she was a toddler in love with nursery rhymes, my younger daughter Katharine rechristened Mother Hubbard Mother Cupboard and so provided me with the heroine of "I Spy Mother Cupboard" and "Mother Cupboard's Dream."

"Looking at Photographs of My Daughters" is for Jessica and Katharine.

The sequence "Everything Is Changed" was written for my sister-in-law, Shirley Wood. The title is the sentence she spoke when her cancer was diagnosed.

"A Walk by the Dugout." For those readers not familiar with Canadian prairie terminology, the dugout here has nothing to do with baseball. It is "a large hole, either shallow or with steep sides, used as a reservoir to catch and hold rain, spring runoff, etc." (See *The Canadian Oxford Dictionary.*)

"Mudra: the Empty Bowl." Mudras are hand gestures or poses associated with both classical Indian dance and yoga meditation. In yoga, the Empty Bowl (one hand cupped in the other, fingers curled up in a bowl-shape) signifies spiritual or psychological emptiness, and waiting for insight.

"Be the River" was written following a workshop on the Don River, given by Austin and Beverly Clarkson and the Milkweed Collective. I thank them for the opportunity to participate. I offer the poem to the Don, in the hope that its mouth may one day be restored.

GHAZALS. Most Canadian poets have come to the ghazal form through John Thompson's powerful collection *Stilt Jack*. I have learned a great deal from Thompson, but was led to him and to the form through Lorna Crozier's "If I Call Stones Blue" in *Everything Arrives at the Light*. Jim Harrison's *Outlyer & Ghazals* deepened my sense of the form's possibilities.

Ghazal 1. Black Elk's statement is taken from *Black Elk Speaks* (University of Nebraska Press, 1979).

Ghazal 3. John Thompson wrote "By tradition, [ghazals] are first of all love poems ..." in an undated manuscript version of his introduction to *Stilt Jack* which I read in Peter Sanger's edition of Thompson's *Collected Poems & Translations* (Goose Lane, 1995). In the published version of the introduction Thompson writes, among other things, "[The ghazal's] order is clandestine."

Ghazal 4. The sentiment, if not the precise words, I've given to Rilke is found in his *Letters to a Young Poet*, translated by Stephen Mitchell (Random House, 1984). John Thompson concludes his introduction to *Stilt Jack* with "The ghazal has been called 'drunken and amatory' and I think it is."

By Any Name. Robert Bly's "Things to Think" is found in *Morning Poems* (Harper Collins, 1998).

Bull's Head Ghazal. The book with the bull's head and the moon on its cover is an edition of Joseph Campbell's *Primitive Mythology*.

Ghazal 8. The third couplet alludes to a couplet from Jim Harrison's "Ghazal 50" in *Outlyers & Ghazals* (in *The Shape of the Journey*, Copper Canyon Press, 1998): "The new marvels of language don't come up from the depths / but from the transparent layer, the soiled skin of things."

Ghazal 9. Kay and Gerda are the two children in Hans Christian Andersen's *The Snow Queen*.

The Drowned Boy poems are for Peter.

ACKNOWLEDGEMENTS

I'm grateful to the University of California Press for permission to reprint various phrases from Gustaf Sobin's "Baby Burials: Domestic Inhumation in the Iron Age," in his essay collection *Luminous Debris*, copyright ©1999 The Regents of the University of California.

Thanks to the editors of the following journals and anthologies who accepted earlier versions of poems for publication; thanks also to the judges who awarded prizes to some of the poems:

The Anthology of New England Writers, v. XI, 1999: "failure to thrive" (Editor's choice, Robert Penn Warren Poetry Award 1999)

Arc: "Bulletins from the Inner World (Ghazal 2)" (Honourable Mention, Poem of the Year Contest, 1998), "The Drowned Boy" (2nd prize, Poem of the Year Contest, 2001), "Be the River" (1st prize, Poem of the Year Contest, 2002)

Contemporary Verse 2: "Twilight," "A Moment's Absence," "Hunger" (2nd prize, Bodies of Water Contest, 1997), "This House Is Full of Longing"

Event: "'Everything Is Changed,'" "Ghazal 4: For the Clover-Strewn Verge"

Ex Libris: "everyone has a life like this"

The Fiddlehead: "Transactions"

Grain: "The Particulars," "Mudra: the Empty Bowl" (2nd prize, 2000 Short Grain Contest, prose poem)

The Malahat: "I Spy Mother Cupboard," "Blue Willow," "Death of a Marlboro Man," "Early Childhood Education"

Poetry Canada: "Flowers for My Mother," "Family Pastimes," "Fear of Knives: the Prairie," "I Must Change My Life: Homage to Rilke"

Room of One's Own: "We Weave Our Lives from Grief and Call It Other Things"

Kitchen Talk: Contemporary Women's Prose and Poetry, edited by Edna Alford and Claire Harris, Red Deer College Press, 1992: "I Spy Mother Cupboard"

Listening with the Ear of the Heart: Writers at St. Peter's, edited by Dave Margoshes and Shelley Sopher, St. Peter's Press, 2003: "A Walk by the Dugout," "Ghazal 3: Name Games at St. Peter's"

Vintage 95, League of Canadian Poets Anthology, 1995: "Looking at Photographs of My Daughters"

Thanks as well to:

Joe Rosenblatt, my first poetry teacher.

Tim Lilburn and the 1995 Sage Hill Fall Poetry Colloquium.

The Ontario Arts Council and Brick Books, Wolsak & Wynn, and *Books In Canada*, for Writers' Reserve grants.

The Saskatchewan Writers Guild Colony Committee, and Colony Coordinators Catherine Macaulay and Shelley Sopher, as well as my fellow colonists, both summer and winter, from 1995 to 2004.

The monks and staff of St. Peter's Abbey and College, at Muenster, Saskatchwan.

Staff and participants in the 1998 Writing Studio at the Banff Centre for the Arts, particularly Don McKay, Sharon Thesen, Roo Borson and Colin Bernhardt.

Irene McGuire, Winston Smith and Susan Folkins of the lamented late Writers & Co Bookstore.

Members of the Friday night Vic poetry group.

Douglas Chambers for friendship, faith in the work and refuge at Stonyground.

Jan Horner for vitally important poetry talk, hospitality and good times.

Ken Howe for elliptical conversation and much-needed laughter.

Beverly and Austin Clarkson and the members of the Milkweed Collective.

Rhea Tregebov for reading and commenting on an earlier version of the MS.

Joan Kaufman for her breathtaking cover photograph and her generous response to the poems.

Barry Dempster, editor *sans pareil*, for his winning combination of tact, assertion and affection. I couldn't have done it without you, Barry.

Beth Follett of Pedlar Press — thanks for your willingness to accept this book and for your excitement about it. Now it's done I hope we'll still have dinner and talk from time to time.

Zab, designer extraordinaire.

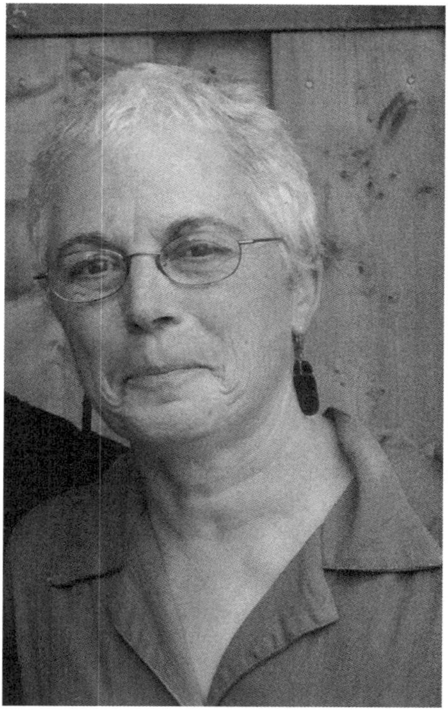

MAUREEN SCOTT HARRIS is a poet and essayist. Born in Prince Rupert, BC, she grew up in Winnipeg and now lives in Toronto, where she works as production manager for Brick Books. Her earlier publications are *A Possible Landscape* (Brick Books, 1993), and the chapbook *The World Speaks* (Junction Books, 2003).